# Axios; Mental Health for the Modern Man

# Axios; Mental Health for the Modern Man

By

Justin A. Mercer

<u>Dedication:</u>

For Christine and Allen, Vivian and Barry, Audrey, Naomie, Wedge and Bronco, Larry, Ethan, Braedy, Jake, Chandler F,  Jeffery, Anna, Chandler B, Conor, Zach, Ben, Safa, Alex, Gus, Sara, Micah, and many others who have walked with me on the journey that got me to a place capable of producing this book. Thank you for being a part of my life and forming my circle.

<u>Foreword:</u>

As a Humanities teacher by trade and training, I know that the title is supposed to read "Axios: Mental Health for the Modern Man".  While I know it does not read that way on the cover for aesthetic purposes, that is the book's title as can be seen on the title page. As I have worked with students as they read through various works and novels, trying to determine why an author made curtains red, or why the house had blue paint... I just wanted to state:  The use of a semicolon in the title is intentional!

The semicolon is a powerful symbol in the world of mental health. As it does in grammar, a semicolon means you paused. You took a breath before continuing. It is not a stop, it does not end a sentence with the finality of a period. It is simply a break before continuing. I experienced a semicolon moment when I held a gun to my head at the age of

18, and I was fortunate enough to pause and think. Not too much about the consequences, I knew what I was intending to do, but more about how I would be discovered, and who would do the discovering. That moment of hesitation, that small pause, was enough to convince me to see the sunrise the next day. That small pause had a ripple effect, and many years later it has led to me feeling fulfilled in life and generally happy with the way it is going. It took hard work, it took setbacks, it took tears, blood, and sweat. It was all worth it.

If life has you in a dark place, this is your call to pause. Who knows what your pause will lead to? You have to be here to find out.

As a further note, this book is targeted towards men and written from the point of view of one. Being a man is my lived experience. While I might use the words guys, men, boys, etc, I fully believe the actionable items in this book are for everyone and I intend for it to be a work of inclusivity. How could I, a man, possibly write "hey, you are a woman and I deeply know and understand the complex societal and social issues you are going through because of your gender, here is how I would solve those problems..." So, I opted not to do that! People of any gender, color, creed, and sexuality are welcome to this book and regardless of your background and why you are here, I hope this book contains something useful to you.

Thanks to Abby Wambach, former player for the USWNT and scorer of 184 goals on the international stage, and her book "Wolfpack" for inspiring that last message of inclusivity.

# Table Of Contents

## Chapter 1: Men's Mental Health- What is the Situation?

The Men of the Western World face a turning point.  By all indicators and studies, the mental health numbers for men are far lower than they are for Women. Women report higher rates of depression, anxiety, and just about every other mental health issue, save for one. Men claim a grisly first place in only one category: Suicide. According to the American Foundation for Suicide Prevention men died at a rate of 3.63x as much as women. Why? How are the numbers for the most drastic thing a person can do higher for men while they have statistically lower serious mental health problems across the board?

To understand the problem requires us to look at the data. Thankfully for us, the Men's Suicide Epidemic is well documented, at least in the United

States. For 2020, the most recent year of CDC and NIH data at the time of writing, suicide was either the 2nd or 3rd leading cause of death for men aged 10-44. The leading cause of death for that age range being Unintentional Injury.  For ages 25-34: 6,882 men died by suicide. For some perspective we can compare the deaths of that age range by suicide, with one of the biggest most disruptive news stories of 2020, if not of the decade: Covid-19. For the same age range, 25-34, of men Covid-19 was responsible for 1,466 deaths. In 2020 a man in their early life was roughly 6x as likely to die by their own hand than by the world-stopping pandemic. This is unacceptable.

Looking a little deeper into the problem, there are many reasons for the suicide numbers of young men to be a leading cause of death. For one, at this stage of life most of our bodies are relatively healthy. You might not be in peak physical condition, but your body is relatively strong. Diseases might keep you down for a week if they are bad, but most often you are not going to be hospitalized by something like the flu, or even Covid-19 if you are in the 10-44 age range barring any underlying conditions.  Even if we have less than healthy habits, it is years before the health effects of things like smoking or having a bad diet become death-causing afflictions. Which is why in the 45-54 age range, heart disease becomes the leading cause of death for men by a long shot, overtaking accidents and pushing suicide and homicide down the list. Physical health is important too.

Okay, so far we have looked at the obvious: the older you get the more likely *something* takes you out. Life will end one day, our job is to arrive at that moment hopefully having lived a life worth living. Now let's deal with the uncomfortable, suicide is the only cause of death that is entirely a choice. Equally, it is the only cause of death that is preventable. Homicide?  Accidents? Yeah, maybe your choices put you somewhere bad, or maybe you were just unlucky. Suicide is not a result of lack of luck. It is a choice. It is a human saying that they would rather face the unknown of after-death and cease their existence than live another day. It is a human being deciding that there is no better way forward, that whatever they are dealing with is so far beyond repair. That is tragic. That is abysmally sad. We owe it to ourselves as a species to do better.

Why do men have such drastically higher suicide numbers than women? Make no mistake, women die by suicide as well, and women are far more likely to attempt suicide than male counterparts. Women have a reporting rate of 1.5x for attempted suicides compared to men according to the American Foundation for Suicide Prevention. Yet men are dying by suicide 3.88x more than women. This data discrepancy bears some looking into.

The discrepancy between reported attempts and completed deaths by suicide for men and women boils down to one key factor: the chosen method of ending one's life. Men are more likely to choose methods that are far more lethal. Firearms accounted for over half of all suicide deaths across the genders in 2020, and its use as a method definitely skews towards men. Jumping from height is another one that skews towards being employed by men. Both of these methods are fairly absolute, and barring miraculously surviving a fall, they are pretty certain in their outcome. The data shows that women typically skew towards less immediate methods of attempting to die by suicide: mainly overdosing on medication or cutting. These methods are lethal, yet often do not act as fast as a bullet or a fall. This gives

time for either the attempter to call for help, or for

outside help to find the struggling person. Regardless

of the method, all attempts should be taken seriously.

Another reason why there is a discrepancy

between reported attempts and number of deaths by

suicides between the genders is another facet of the

methods chosen. If someone holds a loaded gun to

their head with every intention of pulling the trigger,

but does not end up pulling the trigger, is that a

suicide attempt? If someone stands on the ledge of a

building, fully intending to jump, but does not, is that

a suicide attempt? According to the National

Institute of Health, it is. A suicide attempt is " a

nonfatal self-directed potentially injurious behavior

with any intent to die as a result of the behavior. A

suicide attempt may or may not result in injury."

Now the odds are if you are in a mental place where

you were so seriously considering ending your life as to hold a weapon to your head or stand on a ledge, then you are probably not in the mental state to go to a hospital following your "aborted attempt" as the professionals call it. Your attempt is therefore not counted in any official data, and even if you seek help later and speak about your attempt with a therapist it will still not be counted. We can extrapolate that attempts at suicide for both men and women are far higher than the official numbers, which in 2018 the US Government believed that 1.4 million adults in the US attempted suicide.

Speaking of numbers, men are also far less likely to seek any external or "official" help for their mental health. This leads to more skewed numbers and data for all of the bean counters out there to scratch their heads at. By the numbers 1 out of every 4 women in the United States, 25% of the female population, have dealt with a diagnosable mental health issue at some point in their life, be it a temporary or long term issue.  The numbers drop considerably for men, where we barely crack 15%. Realistically men should be on par with women in this category.

Clearly, we have a problem. There are an exorbitant number of self inflicted deaths in the United States, and many of those are our young men who are supposed to be in the prime of their life. Men are dying by suicide at incredibly high rates while both maintaining numbers that state men are less affected by mental health problems overall and attempt suicide at a lower rate. The common denominator? Well, it is us, Men. We both have and are the problem. Let's explore ways to fix it.

## Chapter 2: Axios; A Mindset from Our Past for Our Present

Axios! One of my favorite Greek phrases to ever be muttered by a Roman general. The story of Axios begins in the Roman Empire under the reign of a certain Emperor Nero. Nero is widely considered to be a bad emperor. He is not a leader that anyone should wish to follow, putting himself and his needs before the needs of his Empire. According to legend, Nero sat on his balcony and played the lyre while a good section of Rome burnt to the ground. Working theory is that he ordered the blaze started himself so that he might have a new palace built where homes and shops used to stand. Enter the story of Axios: a Greek affirmation meaning "I am worthy."

The real story of Axios begins with General Gnaeus Corbulo, a man who rose to prominence in the early Roman Empire under Emperor Claudius in the late 40s CE by putting down revolts by Germanic people near modern Cologne. Corbulo gained a reputation as someone who could get things done. He was granted growing responsibility and proved to be successful at every turn. His soldiers loved working for him, as he was both a fair and brilliant commander. Succeeding in battle after battle, and making sure to look after the welfare of his soldiers. After the death of Emperor Claudius; the new emperor, Nero, would also place his trust in General Corbulo.

Nero sent Corbulo to wrangle with the eastern part of the Roman Empire. This is an area we would know as modern day Armenia, Syria, Turkey, Lebanon, Israel, Jordan, even down into Iraq. Corbulo spent much of his time in the east battling the neighboring Parthian Empire, and attempting to overcome incompetence by former Roman commanders in the region. With victory after victory, including some won without bloodshed, Corbulo proved his worth as a general time and again. His soldiers respected him and would march into hell for him. He even gained a popular following back in Rome, where the wealthy and powerful began speaking his praises around their tables.

The same could not be said of Emperor Nero, who was considered a tyrant by the upper class of Rome. On top of the whole fiasco with the fire in Rome, Nero freely spent the money of other aristocrats, and he was also  fond of mutilating and burning people alive who crossed him in many ways. . Nero created many enemies and had survived assassination attempts, leading to him being rightfully afraid of outright rebellion.

Unfortunately for General Corbulo, one of the conspirators against Emperor Nero was Corbulo's son in law. This betrayal by a family member of Corbulo was  coupled with Nero's fear of Corbulo for his popularity with both the common people and with the upper class. As far as historians can tell, Corbulo never actively participated in any plot to make himself Emperor, but he would have been a very popular choice had Nero fallen.

Nero, afraid for his reign, ordered Corbulo to return to Rome from the east, sending another general named Vespasian to take over his command in Judaea.

Along the way, Nero had General Corbulo intercepted en route to Rome in the city of Corinth, a port in Roman controlled Greece. Nero's messengers demanded Corbulo answer for his supposed and unfounded desire to become Emperor by taking his own life. Corbulo, ever the servant of Rome and probably wanting to avoid the horrors he had seen Nero inflict on people who angered him, agreed to do just that. However, his sacrifice for Rome came with a twist. As Corbulo ended his own life, he is reported to have shouted "Axios!" I am worthy.

With that shout, Corbulo defied an Emperor and declared that he himself knew he was far more worthy of ruling Rome than Nero. As an important footnote to the story, it would not be long before Nero was overthrown. There was a brief time of turmoil during the Year of Four Emperors, but the winner of that Game of Thrones style fight and the next long serving Emperor was the man Nero had sent to replace Corbulo: Vespasian.

There are many lessons we can take from the story of Axios. We can look at the leadership qualities of both Corbulo and Nero, realizing that good leaders provide an example and are willing to actually lead. Where bad leaders order and attempt to rule through fear.  Aside from its points on leadership, this  tale has a twofold message in regards to mental health. The first part is cautionary: don't give in to the tyrant trying to rule your life. Corbulo proved to be too proud and too ensnared by the idea of the Emperor, that he did not seek to remove the sickness that was plaguing himself and Rome. The unfortunate truth is that Corbulo could have easily raised his armies and marched on Nero, he just chose to not seek help and counsel to do so. Sometimes it feels like your own mental health problems are a tyrant that is ruling over your life. It clouds your decisions, backs you into corners, and makes you think there is no way out. Pointing to the story of Corbulo, he was under similar pressure, but had options that he refused to recognize. Just as we all have armies of people, known and unknown who would come to our aid if called upon. Remember to call on them.

The other side to this story is to remember that you ARE worthy. It might take a herculean effort to overcome your inner tyrant, but know that you are worthy of the life you desire. At the end, Corbulo understood that he would have made a far better emperor than Nero. He was worthy of living. He was worthy of being Emperor. He was worthy of having the support of Rome. Just as YOU are worthy. YOU are worthy of happiness, of love, of support. You are worthy of building your success, of overcoming your trials. You are worthy of the good in the world. You are worthy of finding peace.

I challenge you to remember Axios. In your darkest moments remember to not give in to the inner tyrant. Remember that you are worthy. Worthy of getting help, worthy of love and respect, worthy of the life you desire. Axios is a mantra that you should be repeating to yourself until you truly believe it. Psychologists would call that "retraining your brain". By believing in Axios, you are believing in yourself. When confronted with a challenge, remind yourself that you are worthy. When facing a setback, remind yourself that you are worthy. You will be amazed by how this mindset from history can help change your present today.

## Chapter 3: Be A Man; Overcoming Modern Social Challenges and "Toxic Masculinity"

It is a phrase that you are probably all too familiar with: Toxic Masculinity. A conversation killer. Probably said by someone to you on the tail end of a rant about how men are bad and how you should feel bad. Well, that is not entirely what the phrase means.

The idea of toxic masculinity implies that there is also non-toxic masculinity. Toxic being something corrosive, poisonous, something bad. Just as having a good hamburger every now and then is perfectly fine and one of the joys of life, it would equally not be good to have a steady diet of Big Macs. This is the meaning of toxic masculinity.  It basically is what happens when someone takes the "Be a Man" song from the classic 90s Disney film *Mulan* far too seriously. Masculinity is not inherently toxic; as most ideas are not inherently toxic. However, if most ideas are taken to an extreme end then they can become dangerous, corrosive, or  poisonous. Either to their adherents or to other outside people. Religion, politics, philosophy, most of us are not fans of extremists about anything. Yet in the case of masculinity we have allowed extremist ideas to invade our societal fabric and pollute the minds and souls of men. Toxic Masculinity is when  men get wrapped up in something "manly" that it becomes corrosive to them and their spirit, and brings others down with them. There is nothing wrong with being a man and enjoying traditional "manly" pursuits. Now with that explanation out of the way, let's explore why toxic masculinity is a detriment to men's mental health.

What does it mean to be a man? Going back to the 90's *Mulan* movie for a moment it means you must be" swift as a coursing river, all the force of a great typhoon, all the strength of a raging fire, and mysterious as the dark side of the moon. Now of course the song describing these traits of what makes a "perfect man" is ironic in its portrayal as the heroine, Mulan, is excelling in these feats secretly alongside her other fellow trainees.

If we look at the song from the lens of men's mental health we can see the traits that at their most extreme define the concept of toxic masculinity. Physical strength compared to angry and destructive forces of nature and encouraging a model man to be "mysterious". Interpret that as silent, never showing anything, especially not emotions. A combination that has seeped its way into our society and is as corrosive to men's souls as battery acid.

Let's tackle the first pillar of manhood espoused in the Mulan song: physical strength. Physical strength is definitely a feature that is valued in the world. We have adored strong men since we first began telling stories. One of the first "superheroes", and one of our first stories that humankind wrote  was the Ancient Sumerian legend of Gilgamesh. A man who fought demons and attempted to conquer death. This fascination with powerful men carried through almost every civilization and some of our greatest legends and real life heroes are known for their strength. This is okay. Physical strength is something that we as men and as a society as a whole should value.  Physical strength allows the firefighter to haul a wounded person from a blazing building, the construction worker to swing his hammer for the thousandth time that day, or the MMA fighter to gain a type of advantage over his opponent. Valuing physical strength is not a problem. However, when taken to the extreme it is something that proves a detriment to men.

How many of you have looked at an advertisement that had a male athlete or model and they were absolutely shredded? Abs that would make Superman or a Greek God jealous, biceps that have to be checked at TSA because they qualify as weapons, shoulders that Atlas wished he had to hold up to the world. Now look at the men around you in your spaces. Your office, your school, your social lives. Probably not many of you. There are definitely very fit men out there, you might even be in this category and probably have many other men in your life who are...but are they as absolutely cut as Cristiano Ronaldo or Conor McGregor? I would hazard a guess and say "no". Just as the persistent images of societal "perfection" displayed in various forms of media weigh on women's minds, it can weigh on men's too.

To the idea of physical strength I say: be you. Be authentically you. Do you want to or need to be a physical specimen? Fantastic, do that. Is the gym not your thing, but are you worried about how others perceive you? Stop that. Be who you are and the right people for you will want to be around you. Regardless, you have to live your life for yourself.

The gym can also be a great tool for helping get control of your mental health, but I would encourage you to be there for intrinsic reasons. The "I want to get physically fit so that I feel better". Not: "I want to get physically fit so that Susie a few desks over notices me". You start taking care of yourself and living your life for you, and not what others think and I am sure people will notice the difference.

This leads to the second part of the song and another pillar of toxic masculinity: be as mysterious as the dark side of the moon. On top of being physically tough, a real man is a mental fortress. Durable, stable, silent, a mystery. Now this narrative is slowly beginning to shift among younger generations and is slowly flowing upwards, but we are not there yet.  As a guy, I feel it is harder for us to be emotionally vulnerable  even despite the progress. I'm not talking being emotional as in having hysterical breakdowns every five minutes. No one wants to deal with that regardless of gender, and if you happen to find yourself in a place where having frequent breakdowns is a problem then I strongly encourage seeking professional help. More on that act later.

Instead I am talking about the societal pressure to be constantly "strong". The cultural need to say "I am okay" even to people who would happily listen if you aren't. The sense that you will be judged for having emotions, that you have to keep your mental anguish quiet to maintain an image of strength.

It is tough admitting fault or talking about something that could be perceived as weakness. We are conditioned that we are in competition with everyone and especially other guys. Competition to be noticed by bosses, by potential mates, hell even by each other to gain social status. Guys frequently talk about themselves as "wolves" and refer to themselves in pseudo-animalistic types by declaring themselves "alphas" or "betas". Not even wolves exist in a life of pure competition, the wolf pack survives by working together. There are leaders and there are followers, but they all work together, pulling in the same direction, to ensure survival of the pack.

Men need to reframe our thinking around our emotions. Having emotions does not equate to weakness. Dealing with emotional issues openly and in a safe environment would actually improve your personal mental fortitude and thereby strengthen your pack. It is time to be "that guy". Be the one to begin speaking up when you are hurt. Have all the strength of a raging fire and open up to your friends. If they are truly your friends then you aren't really walking out onto too much of a ledge. If they don't respond well to one of their own dealing with some stuff, then maybe they are not the crowd you need, not the pack you should run with, and not the circle you should keep.  You might even find yourself being a hero to someone else who has been aching for a signal that it is okay to discuss their feelings. By being the first to take that leap of faith, you are being a leader. You are paving the way for healthier and more real relationships between you and your friends.

I firmly believe that people are stronger together. Be authentically you to your circle, group, crew, tribe, pack,brotherhood, whatever you want to call them. The good ones will have your back and you might end up helping someone else in your circle by taking that brave first step. The key to being a real man of strength and living a rewarding life is to be authentically you. This is how we overcome the entrapments of "toxic masculinity". We recognize the problem and speak power into those who are working to overcome it. By tearing down some of these ridiculous expectations for men, we can begin to shape a better landscape for men's mental health.

# Chapter 4: Telling Your Story: A Societal Antidepressant

"There is no greater agony than bearing an untold story inside of you"

The above quote, from *I Know Why the Caged Bird Sings* by Maya Angelou is true today, tomorrow, and a thousand years ago. Being able to tell your story is liberating and in many cases it can act as its own anti-depressant. Having someone to talk to is part of the concept behind therapy. Speaking our stories allows us to connect with people, we are after all social creatures. "Your story" does not even have to be a tragic tale, or a deep life talk. Even just talking about how your day has gone with someone can bring relief.

To understand the significance of storytelling and its role in our society, I want to once again look to our past. Let me take you back to the old land of Mesopotamia and the city of Baghdad. Now if you are a child of the 80s or 90s and earlier, you might remember Baghdad and its appearances on CNN through the lenses of the Gulf War and Operation Iraqi Freedom. Maybe you or a family member served in one of those conflicts, or have family from the Middle East that was affected by those wars. What we in the Western world all saw on CNN and the despotic and ill-run regime of Saddam Hussein is not representative of the history of that ancient city. For the sake of this story, let's go even further back to the mid-late 700s when a man named Harun Al-Rashid was Caliph of the Islamic Empire, with its capital in Baghdad.

In the late 700s the religion of Islam was synonymous with an empire ruled by the Abbasid Caliphs. One of the most notable of these leaders was a man by the name of Harun Al Rashid. Harun would preside over a time considered to be the start of the

Islamic Golden Age. While religion obviously played a large part in the life of Baghdad and Harun's empire, it was also a city and empire of science, culture, and commerce. There were not many cities as advanced as Baghdad in the 700s. Rome had fallen, Europe was in the Dark Ages, Constantinople was in its very long decline. The Islamic world was at the forefront of science, culture, mathematics, and all the things we care about in modern society. Leading his people through the start of this great golden age was Harun Al-Rashid.

Harun is a very real king, and his historical accomplishments would give him the title "The Great" if he were from Greece or Rome,  but he also appears as a fictionalized character in the stories of *1001 Arabian Nights*. While the anthology is far older than Harun, it had been passed down in oral tradition and was not compiled into written work until after his death. For those who are not familiar

with the stories, *1001 Arabian Nights* is a

compilation of stories told by a woman named

Scheherazade to her husband who is a king. She tells

these compelling stories to prolong her life as the

king won't kill her as he is enthralled with the stories.

The king suffers from depression having been

slighted by his first wife and has vowed to only

remain married to any one woman for a day before

killing her and sparing himself the pain of betrayal. A

truly drastic measure to never feel heartbreak again.

Scheherazade was the daughter of the king's vizier,

and when her turn was called to be married to the

king for a day, she was determined to not go quietly

into the night.  She invites her younger sister, who is

doomed to marry the king the next day, to hear one

last bedtime story before the king has her killed.

Scheherazade is clever, and leaves her first story on a

cliffhanger, enticing the king to prolong her life so that he might hear the next part of the story, sparing Scheherazade until the next night. On and on it goes night after night as Scheherazade weaves these magnificent stories, always ensuring she ends on a cliffhanger so that the king wishes to hear what happens the next night.  These mythical and enchanting stories were told and retold throughout the Middle East and India until finally being written down...and even then still added to. Some of your favorites and ones you have probably heard of like Sinbad and Aladdin were not added until much later.

In one of these stories told by Scheherazade to her husband, the great king Harun Al-Rashid asks his royal vizier, a man by the name of Jafar, for advice as he feels weighed down. Quoting the story: "The sultan said, 'I have taken up in my fingers and let fall all the jewels of my treasury; the rubies, the emeralds, and the sapphires, but not one of them lifted my soul to pleasure. I have been to my harem and passed in review the white and the brown, the copper colored and the dark, but none of them lifted my soul to gladness. I went to my stables, but not one of my countless horses could amuse me, and the veil of the world has not lifted.'"

Harun has taken in all of the earthly pleasures that a king could possibly have: his money, his transportation, his women, and he still feels a great weight on his heart. His advisor is thoughtful for a moment, then suggests that the king disguise himself, go forth from the palace, and seek out the stories of his people. Jafar also disguises himself and accompanies his king on this journey of self discovery.  Harun Al-Rashid makes his way through Baghdad, listening to stories his people tell and with each connection made, he begins to feel better bit by bit. The act of hearing people speak their stories and being able to be open about his own helped this mighty and powerful king overcome his depression.

Sneakily, the original storyteller, Scheherazade, was trying to tell the story of Harun-Al Rashid to her king so that he would listen to more stories and be cured of his depression, hopefully sparing her life in return. A story about curing depression within a story about curing depression. Worthy of a Leonardo Dicaprio film.

The advice of Scheherazade/Jafar given to their respective kings is sound and echoes true throughout time and language. True human connection, listening to others and hearing their stories. This is a path to happiness that no amount of jewels or horses or the size of your harem can compete with. We are social creatures who do better forming real connections, not marriages of a single day.

To this point, I encourage finding real connection. Find a group of people who you can become invested in and that are willing to become invested in you. Listen to their stories and share yours.  These people will become your circle, your system of support, your way of breaking out from behind the veil over your life, maybe you already have this group, maybe you are in the process of seeking them out.  This advice worked for ancient kings, and it can work for men and women of today. You never know what stories you might hear and how they can help you. On the other side of the same token: don't be afraid to tell your story. You never know who might need to hear it.

Sharing our stories gives us a power we can scarcely imagine. By furthering and deepening our relationships with others we help build a solid foundation for ourselves. Encouraging real human connection in all aspects of our lives works to lift us all up. A rising tide raises all ships.

# Part Two: Mental Health in Your Personal Life

So far we have looked at some overarching societal ways we can improve men's mental health. Mainly encouraging a culture where men believe they are worthy, tearing down corrosive and toxic elements that seek to drive men apart and make them feel unworthy, and by encouraging a sharing of our stories; so that we might form better, deeper, and more real connections with people around us. This all calls for a cultural shift that can begin in your offices, schools, shops, and homes. To be in a place to take charge and lead a cultural shift takes being personally secure in yourself. It is a taxing thing to put yourself out there and to tell your story. It is downright draining to build a supportive network of people throughout your life. This work can take a lot out of you.

To affect real change outside ourselves we must first be on the journey to bettering our own personal lives. Figuring out how to handle our personal struggles, the demons that haunt us. While building a better society is both noble and necessary, you would not want to lead a half starved and ill-equipped army to war, nor would anyone want to follow a commander who was ill-prepared to lead.

While we all struggle, and I know I personally continue to struggle with mental health, it is important to be making a real effort to move the needle in your own mind. A real leader is willing to do the work that they ask others to do. If you are not willing to work on yourself, how can you expect others to work on themselves to build the better society for men's mental health that we talked about? You can't. With this in mind, the rest of this book will look at mental health in our own lives so that we might better understand ourselves and put our own selves on a path to healing. As airlines frequently say "when the oxygen masks fall, put your own mask on before assisting others". This directive works just as well and for the same reasons with mental health as it does with oxygen flow during an airborne emergency.

## Chapter 5: Fear is the Path to the Dark Side

A wise Kermit the Frog sounding Jedi Master once said: "Fear is the Path to the Dark Side. Fear leads to Anger. Anger leads to Hate. Hate...leads to Suffering." This saying is one of the most powerful ones to come out of the Star Wars universe in my humble opinion. Star Wars is a fascinating universe, one where ancient Chinese philosophy meets King Arthur and adds a splash of turbolaser fire. George Lucas created a powerful and enduring universe, and even though the prequel movies might be less than loved by some fans, I thank them for giving us lines like the one Master Yoda spoke above.

I grew up with Star Wars. Before I knew enough to understand movies at all, my dad held me as I watched X-wings careen down the Death Star trench.  When I was hardly five, my dad took me to see *A Phantom Menace* in theaters on opening weekend. My childhood was surrounded by TIE fighters, lightsabers, and re-enacting fight scenes with my father. Like many young men and women from the 1970s onward, Star Wars has become a part of my life.

The beauty of the "Fear leads to Anger" saying is that it can be applied to so many wildly different situations and scenarios and still hold true. I want to apply this phrase to mental health and the decision to take healthy but tough steps to confront those issues, or not. To do that, I will share a bit about my journey down the path to the Dark Side in hopes that my story can shed some light on actions that should be taken, and definitely on actions that should not be taken.

Fear is a powerful motivator. A healthy dose of fear kept your ancient ancestor's head on a swivel and allowed them to see that saber toothed tiger sneaking up on them. A healthy dose of fear probably kept you alive at some point in your life. Be it from taking an extra second to see that semi truck barreling towards you before pulling out into the road, being alert enough to see an attacker waiting to jump you down that dark alley, or many other scenarios. Fear is a useful tool. It can make us stop, think and survey a potentially dangerous situation, and it can supercharge our reactions allowing us to fight or flee our way out of equally dangerous scenarios. Fear also has a nasty habit of gripping us at the wrong times in the wrong ways.

On my personal mental health journey I noticed pretty quickly that I was afraid to tell people pretty much anything. Personal stories, feelings, hell even what brand of t-shirt I liked. I was so anxious about being seen as an "other" that I distinctly remember in high school asking my mother to buy me clothing with no labels so that other kids would have less of an avenue to make fun of me about something. I was in a constant state of fear. Anxiety compounded by assholes is never a fun mix.

I was afraid that my experience: one of profound and pervasive unhappiness no matter what "good" things happened, was normal, and if it is normal then why would anyone want to hear about it? Boo hoo suck it up. Then I was afraid that if my experience was not normal, then I would be judged by friends and family or by those who would seek to use such knowledge against me. That I would be perceived as weak for feeling a certain way. Everyone else seemed to have such normal and happy lives, so I was afraid to let it be known that I did not fit that mold. At this point in my life I had no idea what depression or anxiety entailed or that I in fact was dealing with that two headed monster. Depression and anxiety were mental illnesses, things that happened to other people and were most definitely not talked about by anyone "normal". I began struggling with these monsters when I was twelve, and I would not have a name for these mental struggles until I was almost nineteen.

Gradually my fear of being rejected or turned away for feeling the way I did turned to anger. I was angry at the world. Why couldn't anyone hear me or see the pain I was in? Well I was playing myself and falling into a trap that is all too common with any mental illness, because if you don't speak, how can anyone hear you? Mostly, I was angry at myself. I was angry about everything I did. From how I could not achieve great things, to how I was struggling to make friends or find a romantic partner. I was angry that I was not as physically fit as I wanted to be no matter how hard I perceived myself trying, angry that I was not enjoying things I thought I should be. Angry that I felt like crap all the time. Angry that I felt deeply unhappy for seemingly no good reason. Angry that I was angry.

Anger quickly turned to hatred. I hated everything I was involved in. Food that I used to enjoy lost its flavor and turned to ash.  Activities and diversions that  I used to love or find solace in no longer provided any respite, and I hated them for it. I was full of hatred for myself and how I was. It was a vicious downward spiraling cycle of being afraid, being angry, and then being full of hate. This was not sustainable. I suffered in my internal anguish, alone. Fear led to Anger, Anger led to Hate, Hate led to Suffering.

This downward spiral of fear, anger, and hatred nearly led to me being dead by suicide, and it all could have been avoided if I had faced my fear at its earliest onset. We have been conditioned to keep our problems to ourselves. When we do speak out, grasping for any sort of hope we are often met with some version of "well X person has it worse than you". You know what? Yeah, there are plenty of people who probably have it worse than you and the same amount that have it better than you. That is life. That does not mean that your problems are not valid.

If you find yourself anywhere on this downward spiral of fear, anger, hatred, and suffering, this is your call to proceed to the nearest exit, keeping in mind that it might be behind you. This is a spiral that is unsustainable. The stress I experienced during my darkest days alone has probably shaved years off of my life. There is help out there. There are good people out there. It is work, and it is downright terrifying when you first admit to someone you have a problem, but overcoming that fear and putting in that work is worth it. It is not instant, there is no

magic button that makes everything happy instantly.

It takes work, and it takes time. Yet it is worth it. It is

necessary. As the same wise Kermit the Frog

sounding Jedi Master also said: "Try not, DO. Or do

not, there is no try."

## Chapter 6: It's Okay to Not Be Okay

I've been fortunate enough to be active in mental health related advocacy work for the better part of a decade. During that time I got to see a myriad of catch phrases work their way through the community. Many of them were cringey things that, while probably coming from a good place, seemed to have been made by sorority girl marketing majors for other sorority girls. While not inherently exclusive, some of these marketing phrases just did not breach barriers into many communities that could have also used some mental health advocacy. For some people mental health and self care are far more than yoga and bubble baths.  Thankfully for all the misfires, the climate is slowly changing and even sometimes  the marketing people hit a grand slam.

In 2017, I attended the Active Minds yearly conference in Washington DC.  Active Minds is a mental health advocacy organization that focuses primarily on college students. I was going as part of a delegation from my graduate school since I had been heavily involved in my local Active Minds chapter through most of college and grad school. At the conference I heard many great talks,  advice, and plans for improving mental health for my age demographic in the United States. All while being bemused that I was one of maybe 50 men out of the hundreds of people at this conference. That sampling of men was fairly diverse, covering every race, sexual preference, hair color, body type, anything you want. This was one of those moments when it truly hit me that we needed more men in mental health.

Aside from my sobering realization about men being included in the march towards better mental health, another revelation I had come out of this conference was a phrase that was one of these marketing grand slams. It was so simple yet elegant and powerful; "It's okay to not be okay."

When asked "hey! How are you doing?" How do you answer? Does your answer change depending on who is asking? Do you answer your close friends with the same detached "I'm okay, thanks" as you would a store clerk making polite conversation? Then you are part of the problem.

This societal double-think of simultaneously wanting to seek real connection and yet throwing up walls and shutting ourselves off came to a head for me in Spring of 2022. In my day job I am a high school history teacher, and as much as I like to think the kids learn something from me, they always manage to teach me the most important things.

I first heard the poem "Drowning Fish" performed as a monologue by one of these high school students in their school's annual acting and music showcase. This student, who usually prefers running all the behind the scenes aspects of the theater, delivered the poem with such power and emotion that I was crying my eyes out by the time the audience erupted in applause, and I truly do not cry at much of anything.  I knew the words were not of her own creation, but she delivered them with the passion and pain of someone either incredibly well versed in the art of performance, or as someone who has lived those words. The Drowning Fish is a story of depression and finding yourself in a dark place, and our poet explaining what he wishes he could say in normal conversation when asked "how are you doing?" The original poet is Rudy Francisco, and he delivers the story fantastically well.

I think the reason the words this high school student brought to life hit me hard for many reasons. While the story told in the poem is uniquely Rudy Francisco's, there are so many things he says that I identified with. Every other line had me sinking into my seat thinking "why are you talking about me?"

"I really want to say that I am not in a good place right now...but that is not a polite answer. So, instead I pretend it is Halloween, I Jack-O-Lantern my face into something acceptable and I tell others ' I'm fine' until it sounds like the truth, but sometimes there is a 'help me' chained to the ankle of an ' I'm doing okay' "...when the student was echoing these words I felt like a knife had cut right through the shroud I sometimes like to hide behind. The "I'm okay's" the "I'm fine's", that were both my armor and my curse. It was like this young lady was talking directly to me. I had even written something eerily similar to this in my first book *Hell Has No Stars* describing my own experience with depression and anxiety. I have spoken about this feeling to friends and therapists. In a couple of lines of slam poetry, I felt like the secret words I tend to hide behind had just been revealed to the audience.

Once I got over my main character syndrome, and settled back into the fact that literally anyone in the world can read about my depression and anxiety, and that I am happier for it and for all of the good it has led to... it became an eye opening experience. Statistically out of an audience of around 100 people, there were probably at least 25 of them forming a cross section of race, gender, political spectrum, nationality, any other descriptor you can think of; and they were all thinking like me. Many of us tend to hide behind the "I'm fine" or "I'm okay" walls that we throw up. In some ways it is easier to hide. What if the person asking does not really want to know? Are they making polite conversation or can they see the anguish and anxiety that I can feel reflecting in my eyes as my face remains as stone cold and blank as I can make it? Can I trust them with my answer?

Both men and women hide behind the "I'm fine" walls. Men typically do it to avoid appearing "weak" and women do it for much the same reasons and to avoid the horrible stereotype of "the emotional woman". We all have built up a concept that the world at large does not care about our problems and would judge us for having them and expressing our internal pain. The "I'm fine" is a curse that we all share , but it is one that we can all work on to overcome.

So far in this book I have talked frequently about having and building a circle, a group of people that you trust that support you and that you support in return. Having your circle is a key part to overcoming the curse of "I'm fine". Having people that you know are able to hear you say "I'm not fine". Being a person that listens and lets someone tell you "I'm not okay". Change starts small. If you and your family and friends adopt open communication and are willing to talk about the scary truths of not being okay, then it will spread. While circles overlap, very rarely are they identical. If you create this culture of honesty and vulnerability among you and your friends, they will pass it to their friends. With a lot of work, we can collectively shift the culture around how we deal with mental health. We can make it okay to not be okay.

# Chapter 7: The Challenges of Daily Life

Life is hard. There are many issues we face that are far outside of our control yet deeply affect our personal lives. An oil conglomerate's decision to raise the cost of a barrel of oil trickles down to you not being able to afford that extra trip to go visit your friends across town. A despot's decision to invade a nation half a world away from your own makes the cost of bread or natural gas go up. So on and so forth. If you are anything like me, the decisions of the elite are far out of reach of ever being in your control. Yet barring some sort of great societal change we have to live with the consequences of what a collection of old people think is the best action. All we can do is try and control our immediate situation. I want to look at some examples of my own anxiety and how that presents or does not present in a few situations. I would also like to look at what you can do to help mitigate any mental health crises for your employees, coworkers or students; people that you interact with on a daily basis.

If you are anything like me then global events are incredibly anxiety inducing. My anxiety would be described as "high functioning" meaning my panic attacks, while very real, are not as visible as some others. I mentally shut down, sometimes I breathe a lot harder, and definitely have very little concept of what is going on around me. Sometimes they are brought on by being in stressful situations, but honestly I handle real world stress pretty well.

Case and point for handling real world immediate stress: my partner and I were going to Yellowstone National Park in California. Beautiful park, I highly recommend it. However we were going in winter and the rental car company had "upgraded" our rental to a 2020 Mustang. Cool! I am a sucker for the Mustang. However, Mustangs are not known for their reliability in snow…which in the mountains in winter was a very real problem.  We ended up hitching a ride with some people we met at our campsite outside the park, they had snow chains and we didn't. Unfortunately the poor girl who was driving had no idea how to drive in the snow. In fairness I don't have much experience either having been born and raised in Georgia and Alabama. My partner lived most of her life in Montana and Illinois though, so she probably should have been driving…well the girl went way too fast, spun out on a patch of ice, and ended up in the ditch. My side of the car was mere inches from a bigass tree, I think a Giant Sequoia, that would have surely put a damper on my day. I was fine. Physically and mentally. I hopped out of the car and began working on the problems with my partner. We made sure no one had any injuries and began working on a solution to get the car out of the snow drift.

Doing a 490 degree spin in a Honda Civic on ice and nearly hitting a tree with my face would probably give most people anxiety. Yet I was fine. Cooly and mostly calmly working the situation and problems to make sure we all got out okay. Now on the other hand, I clearly remember a time when I had an anxiety attack for literally no good reason.

It was in my graduate school days and I had just been invited over for drinks by this girl I knew. A couple drinks, a lot of flirting, and before you know it, one thing led to another and I had an anxiety attack...R.I.P my game.  My anxiety was not even about the moment or any of the things happening in my present...but about stupid Russia. At that time, there were lots of news stories about how Russia was gearing up for war, buzzing US aircraft carriers, and how they were planning to expand on their invasion of Crimea. This was 2017. I don't know why, but I was fully convinced at that moment that we were going to have a nuclear exchange, and this overwhelming out of my control stressor caused an anxiety attack when I should have been much more focused on other far more pleasant things happening in the moment. Thankfully the girl was incredibly understanding as she revealed she suffered from anxiety too. Sometimes it takes a moment of incredible vulnerability to have a real connection. We spent the rest of the evening talking about mental health and having a genuine great time and connection. While we realized we were not meant for each other in that regard, we remained friends long after this moment.

In my professional life I have often continued to complete tasks and carry on despite having an anxiety attack. As I have mentioned before; I am a teacher. This means I have an audience almost all of the time during working hours. This makes having an anxiety attack during the workday highly inconvenient. Yet, I have learned how to live with it. If I ever needed a minute outside of my classroom, I was fortunate enough to have colleagues who would not hesitate to watch the kids for a few minutes.

I tell  these stories to make clear that there is no formula for how anxiety presents itself. There is no formula for how any mental illness presents itself. While many of the causes and symptoms have recognizable trends across people, their version of what they struggle with can be just as unique as they are.  On my worst days my depression or anxiety absolutely cuts me down and I am inoperable as a human. Blessedly that has become very rare since I have actively been taking steps to work on my mental health. Some days it renders me less useful, and I have learned to become okay with that. You do not always need to be operating at 100% capacity. It is the same as if you had a cold. You can probably safely do your job, but is that spreadsheet going to get done as fast? Are your phone calls going to be as cheery and upbeat? Probably not.

I would encourage all people in positions of power or authority over others to try and accommodate with empathy as best you can your charges' mental health problems. Most people's lives are spent at work, governed and at the whim of someone else.  For the early part of your life you are in school, also at the whim of others.  Many organizations and corporations pay lip service to employee mental health. I challenge all of them to do better. Your human capital is your business' best resource. The people who work for you are the ones who make your company move forward. Treating them with respect and doing your best to create an environment that these people want to be in will keep them around longer.

I hear people decry the fact that "workers have no loyalty anymore". Well workers don't have loyalty because why would we? Many places feel it is okay to underpay and over manage and over work their employees, yet they are in shock when their employees flee for better opportunities. Things that are often outside of our control apply the most stress and your job is no different. Except your job is how you afford to live life, making its security even more stressful.

For managers, bosses, and educators building an environment where all of your workers/student's mental health needs are met should be a priority. Do you talk about self-care? Well then actually give your employees/students time to take care of themselves. Is your employee working late into the night because of some sort of pressure? Take an honest look at yourself and your company. Does the task they are working on absolutely need to be done right now? No? Tell them. Actively encourage your employees to take breaks. Also, set an example if you are in a position to do so. Take your vacation time, create solid work-life boundaries, be open to constructive feedback and criticism. Your employees, colleagues, or students will learn from your example. Changing your own habits can help change a culture, which in turn can make a healthier and more balanced life for everyone in your sphere of influence. Life is a challenge, but you can make yours and others better.

# Chapter 8: Self-Defeatism: Overcoming Your Worst Enemy

In the battle to grapple with your mental illness, you are your own worst enemy. No one looks at a person with depression, bipolar, schizophrenia and says "I hope they fail". In terms of mental illness, we are often our own biggest obstacle.  To look further into this issue, I offer a quote from Napoleon Bonaparte, the infamous French conqueror: "God fights on the side with the best artillery".

I want to look at this quote from the iconic French Emperor because he is a subject matter expert on defeating an enemy. This is a man who became an Emperor in a place that had just sworn off monarchy in a violent revolution. A man who oversaw the destruction of the Holy Roman Empire, an entity that had existed since the 800s AD/CE, which was around for about five times as long as the United States has existed. His influence would extend from Madrid to Moscow, and his Grand Army would be the most effective fighting force in Europe for a time. He has an impressive resume as both a ruler and commander, and his quip about artillery still holds up to scrutiny if we give the man some creative leeway when it comes to modern technology like aviation and cruise missiles.  Napoleon was skilled at defeating other armies on a field of battle, and as his quote implies, he frequently had the best artillery. As a historian and now history teacher by trade, I often think of the quotes of the "great" people that have come before me. Sometimes I attempt to apply advice given by Napoleon, Julius Caesar, Marcus Aurelius, Teddy Roosevelt, Sun Tzu or other historical figures to my own life. These were wildly successful men, and what they say deserves to be looked at and some of it remembered.  In the case of this Napoleon quote, I find myself struggling to apply it to my life for multiple reasons.  The first glaring one being that I am not an artillery officer...though it does sort of come in handy when I am wearing my soccer coach hat! As one of my co-coaches says to our players "just pepper their goal! One of them is bound to go in!" The other reason is I feel that most of my struggles are internal against anxiety and depression. So, how can I equip myself with the best artillery?

One of my biggest internal enemies is self-defeatism. Self-defeatism is a symptom of my years of dealing with unchecked depression.  Years of believing that wicked voice in my head that does nothing but sow doubt and discord. The voice that tells myself I am not smart enough, good enough, strong enough, good looking enough, man enough. I beat myself in any situation before I ever take the field, court, stage, controller, or any other arena of performance or competition. In these situations, I have shot myself with my own artillery before ever exposing myself to the shots taken by the "enemy".

I imagine most of us have been there before, thinking and saying things such as "I can't" or "No, it is just not possible" or "There is no way this goes well" or "maybe this works for some people, but it is probably not going to work for me" or " I am not worthy".  In this, I know I am not alone. Many men face feelings of inadequacy, of not being enough, of not being worthy. Spend enough time on Reddit and you are bound to see some stories of a guy who probably describes himself as a loser and his story of why nothing is going right.

Our internal self defeatism leads to many outwardly bad things. Some say this is the root of violence, you can point to it as a cause for self harm,

and in a general sense it just makes us miserable to
be around.  In 2022 when this book was written,
there has been a lot of attention towards
"movements" of men who feel alienated by society.
Men who feel that they don't belong. Unfortunately
many of these men are driven to violence, sometimes
it is caused by external people goading them on.
Sometimes people are just not good people and are
predisposed to violence anyway. This violence has
come across against women, people of races different
from their own, and people of creeds different from
their own.

Now this is <u>NO</u> excuse for any sort of violence,
but I would hazard a guess that many of those men
suffer from some kind of mental health problem that
goes unhelped and gets taken advantage of  by other
toxic and downright evil people. At the end of the
day, our decisions are our own, but we should

acknowledge the forces that push people further down incredibly dark paths.

How do we stop all this? The constant bombardment of negative artillery from both internal and external forces? We need to train men to shoot back, figuratively speaking. Psychologists would call this action retraining your brain, or metacognition. Thinking about your thoughts, unpacking them, working through them and telling yourself that the knee-jerk thought of inadequacy that your brain produced after years of conditioning is wrong. It is hard work and it is constant work. You have to be on guard and actively work to stop negative thoughts, break them down, and essentially call yourself out on your own BS.

I prefer the visualization of shooting back. I imagine a line of cannons arrayed on a Napoleonic battlefield unloading walls of fire towards my negativity. You never lost the war when you grew up imagining yourself as a commander, right? So why would you lose this one? My brain wants to shoot some incredibly negative thoughts at me? Well let me fire back. 1800s battlefields not your thing? You can imagine any scenario you wish; a type of sport, a race, a poll, whatever floats your boat. Imagination of a scenario is not required for metacognition, but I have found that the addition of a "winning" thought helps the impact of disassembling your negative ones.

Let me once again stress that this is a lot of work, and it is hard. You have to actively think about the negative thoughts when they try to break through, being on your guard at all times and especially in situations where you are predisposed to believe your own crap. It is work that does not always succeed. A goalkeeper can't possibly keep every shot out of their goal. A pitcher can't throw no-hitters every single game. Not every sales pitch goes swimmingly. The same goes for metacognition, and it is important to realize, much like a goalkeeper, pitcher, or salesman; that messing up is okay. It is going to happen. What is important is that you get back out there and stop that next shot, strike out the next one, or clinch that next sale.

If metacognition seems overwhelming, start small. Take one negative thought you have and begin to unpack it. For example: "I can't do this"...well why not? "This thing is hard" yeah, but I have all these examples of how I have overcome hard things before "Those are different" are they really? Yeah I might not have done THIS thing before, but I have done many things and some of those were great challenges and accomplishments and I am still here, maybe I can do this thing. You don't even have to get yourself to a fully positive answer all the time, just enough to break the cycle of corrosive negativity and spur some belief in yourself.

As Napoleon said, "God fights on the side with the best artillery." When it comes to your brain, self defeatism, and your own cycle of negativity, you have to follow Napoleon's advice. Get your mental artillery on your side. Help others to get their cannons working for them too. Self-defeatism is your worst enemy on any sort of mental or physical health journey. Don't put up with your own crap any more.

# Chapter 9: Find Your Lightning

When you hit rock bottom there is nowhere else to go but up, an oft repeated phrase that is far easier said than done. There might be "nowhere left to go but up"...or you could drag along the bottom for a while. Just because you hit the bottom does not mean you bounce off of it.  It is a moment that we are all probably too familiar with. One thing after another has gone down in flames, you have lurched from tragedy to tragedy with no end in sight. Maybe this long train of hurt has been happening for years, maybe months, hell it could even only take a few days. At this point you find yourself asking for "it" to hit you. To strike you down. God, a storm, the cosmic energy of the universe, whatever you desire "it" to be. Throw one more problem your way. Why not? It becomes some sort of dark comedy. The universe has apparently never held back before. In a cry of frustration, anguish, and pain you ask it to strike you down, as what else could possibly go wrong?

To help us understand finding our lightning, I want to use an example from popular culture. Enter the story of Prince Zuko. As a young boy, Zuko lost his mother and was summarily abused by his father. His father also happens to be a tyrannical ruler of a warlike nation that has committed numerous war crimes; including genocide. From a young age, Zuko was trained in the ways of the warrior. Honor was everything to the young prince. Unfortunately for Zuko, he dishonored his father in his early teenage years by suggesting the lives of soldiers were worth more than being pawns on a battlefield during a war council meeting. His father became enraged at the apparent disrespect and challenged his teenage son to a duel. The older and far more experienced warrior won, horribly maiming his son. As Zuko had refused to fight his father, he was banished from the empire for cowardice. This was a major plot of the kids show *Avatar:The Last Airbender* that aired on Nickelodeon in the 2000s. Yes, a kids show.

Avatar is one of my all time favorite tv shows. I respect the storytelling and how the writers manage to tie in some very adult and real world themes into a story that is digestible for young kids. This show features many situations and scenarios where the young protagonists have to make incredibly adult decisions. It also shows them still trying to be kids and teens and live their lives amid the backdrop of a horrible war and complicated geopolitics, having deep philosophical discussions about the human condition,  all while having the fantasy aspect of learning to master one of the four base elements: water, earth, fire, or air.

At one point in the Avatar story we find Prince Zuko, the banished prince who is struggling to find who he truly is and what his destiny is, standing atop a plateau yelling with unbridled anger. Zuko had just fought off an attack by his sister, a powerful firebender who can control and shoot lightning. Aside from showcasing some not-good family dynamics, the fight shows that  Zuko is not nearly as talented of a firebender. During the fight, Zuko's uncle and guardian was injured. Iroh, Zuko's uncle does turn out to be okay, but the encounter shakes up Zuko. Iroh is the only one who cares about him, and Zuko is terrified of losing him. Zuko begged Iroh to show him how to control and redirect lightning, since Iroh is a master of firebending, he can control and shoot lightning at will. Iroh shows Zuko the correct form and motions to redirect lightning, but categorically refuses to shoot lightning at his beloved nephew to let him practice for real, as it is far too dangerous. In frustration and rage pent up after years of suffering and being denied this one last thing; Zuko takes off to find his own lightning.

Standing atop the plateau as lightning crackles all around him, Zuko begs the universe to hit him. It has thrown everything at him before and never held back, why stop now? Why stop now when he might finally have a tool to hurl some of it back? This scene of frustration is one that is all too familiar for many people. You are upset, angry, frustrated. Life has given you more than you really want to handle, and you find yourself hoping perversely for something else to go wrong, but maybe this time it is something that you can solve, just for the chance to come out ahead on something.

I personally believe that this idea of "yelling at the lightning" in the case of Prince Zuko is a concept we can all take and apply to our own mental health and life journeys. Many people find themselves at the end of a dark tunnel with an insurmountable list of tasks and problems. Things to fix and repair, things to do, things we would rather not do. Accomplishing any sort of meaningful task is compounded in difficulty when we throw in a mental health problem. Your need to continue living life and doing the basic things needed to feed yourself and keep a roof over your head become really hard to do. Continuing to struggle often leads men down darker paths such as alcohol abuse or as previously discussed: violence.

Keeping everything pent up and it will burn through you like a fire. The climb off of rock bottom is slow and tough, but doable. Find your lightning, find that one thing that you can do today. To get yourself off the couch or out of bed, to break you out of that downward slide. It can be something as small

as taking a shower, getting yourself good warm food,
going outside. It can be a bigger thing too: cleaning
the house, changing your oil, applying for that job. It
might be a slide down to the bottom, but it is a climb
back up.

Nothing comes quickly in terms of finding
peace and overcoming your mental health challenges.
Finding your "lightning" , some small thing you can
do to prove to yourself that you are in control can
help immensely if you are at rock bottom, or
somewhere on the slide down.

## Chapter 10 : Hope; Everything in Moderation

As previously mentioned in this book, I love Star Wars. Sometimes when I am under immense stress or just need to decompress, I will throw on one of the movies. It is something familiar, safe, and entertaining. I am sure you have some movie, book, series, or whatever that is the same for you. Recently, the Star Wars spinoff, "Rogue One", has been my go to movie for this.

During my last watch through of this movie I became hung up on one of the seminal lines "We have Hope! Rebellions are built on hope!" It seems a straightforward enough line: where protagonist Jyn Erso proves she has learned the true meaning of why the rebels must fight from her begrudging companion turned ally Cassian Andor as he smiles on while she delivers an impassioned speech to the assembled commanders of the Rebel Alliance. A truly great scene in a movie full of them.

This last watch through, this line provoked some deeper thoughts. I happened to be in the midst of writing an article for my blog: *Average Joe's Mental Health*. I was in a dry spell of creativity and had no idea what to write about. After some conversations with my father, who is also an author, he suggested that I should talk about hope. Simple, effective, timely.

On this watch through of Rogue One, and having already primed to be thinking about hope, this line caused me to reflect on some of my lived experiences. The first being much like Jyn Erso was describing; Where hope was the only thing to cling to. The second being from a much less Disney-like side of life where there was no hope to be had. Two very different experiences in two very different frames of mind.

As I have mentioned a few times throughout this book, I am a teacher for my day job. Teaching is interesting, because unlike most jobs, I am "locked in" to a position for a year. Sometimes with drastic consequences should you choose to pull out of a contract mid year. These can range from losing your license and being blacklisted in certain states, to in my case, my employer was responsible for my housing. Oftentimes you have to make it known months in advance that you do not intend to return the following year. Still being employed through the end of the school year, but casting off stability while you hope you find something new.  This leaves a narrow window for teachers to switch jobs, be it to other schools or out of the education field entirely.

Job hunts are stressful regardless of your situation. Interviews with people that don't matter, personality profiles, computers reading your resumes for keywords so that hopefully you might get your documents seen by a person. Much like online dating, it is very impersonal and can lead to feelings of great inadequacy.

Job after job sent me canned replies: "we have chosen to pursue other candidates at this time" or worse ghosted me after multiple interactions.  Maybe we should simplify job searches to by using something like Tinder. Swipe right if interested, swipe left if not. It would at least make the rejections and ghosting seem more appropriate. It is soul crushing, especially if you feel you meet the qualifications. Why not me? What am I doing wrong? Hope is a tough thing to hold onto when you are faced with setback after setback, false hope after false hope.

In this case, holding onto hope proved useful and allowed me to persevere. I believed there had to be something out there for me in a place I wanted to be. After applying to 100s of jobs, I finally applied to the right one. They were interested in me as a candidate, and I was interested in their project and mission.  Having hope proved useful. It kept me going, kept me searching with some positivity. In my case it proved very useful having a circle of people around me to help keep the belief alive. My very own scrappy group of rebels willing to fight the evil Empire. The rebellion that was built on hope.

The second situation stirred to mind by the proclamation of "rebellions are built on hope" is  one where I had no hope. How can you build anything on hope when it does not exist?  I was deep in the throes of untreated and undiagnosed depression in months leading up to a suicide attempt. I felt isolated and alone, like I was trapped in a prison and could not escape. There were other humans around me as I was at college at the time, but I felt alone and empty. Even in the most crowded of freshman lecture halls.

When you are laying alone in your single dorm room that was designed and built by the same lovely people who built asylums in the 60s and 70s, your surroundings mirror your internal turmoil. Bright fluorescent lights that provide no warmth or comfort matched perfectly with how my brain and soul felt. The lights are on and we are purely functional. The paint peeling from the walls, the years old grime in the corners, the cold tile floors. Everything matched how I felt. Cold, empty, falling apart. There was no hope to be had in that sick, cold, sterile place.

That lack of hope led to a suicide attempt in April 2013. I was 18 years old and had no desire to see 19. Thankfully I was unsuccessful, and even more thankfully, I had people rally around to ensure that would never happen again.

Bringing this back to a more present day me: I was talking my dad's ear off about "I hope I will get this job" and "I hope this" and "I hope that". Basically talking myself in a circle that fluctuated between agonizing concern and a brief fluttering of ill-founded hope, right back to excruciating anxiety over it all. I like to think I have a pretty good brain, but when the anxiety takes hold it can be hard to break it out of its negative pattern or my propensity to just continue talking about the thing giving me anxiety. I was going through this cycle and my father said : "son, hope is not a plan."

I was floored. Such a simple and easy "well no shit, Dad!" phrase and it caught me completely off guard.  Over the last few weeks I have had a chance to unpack this statement and I think my father hit the nail on the head by tying together a few concepts I have struggled with putting into words. My mental health journey has been battling the twin headed demon of anxiety and depression and as I know anyone who has to deal with anything similar can attest, it is an exhausting battle. As many people with depression do, I struggle with being hopeful for the future. It's kind of hard to be hopeful for an abstract better time when your brain is fighting against you and telling you everything sucks. That you are in this dark pit, you are always going to be there, and you can't do anything to get out.

I've found that by having something concrete to work towards, a very real goal with manageable steps to begin shuffling forwards, that I do far better mentally than with the abstract and ill defined ideas of simply hoping and believing. It is tough to hope or believe when your brain is wired to scream the exact opposite. "Nothing works, why would you believe this to be different?" It is a weird feeling knowing your mind is actively sabotaging yourself. Things have obviously worked out okay for me! I live in a time where the standard of living for a majority of the world is far better than it ever has been, and further I am fortunate to be educated, not wanting for food, and fairly certain I will have a roof over my head at night. Yet my brain likes to make me think and feel that everything is going to fall apart at any given time. Walking a tightrope of what I know to be true, and what the anxiety and depression wants me to believe. For me, the biggest anti-anxiety and anti-depressant I get undeniable evidence that something is working. That a plan is coming together and being acted on.

My Dad was just telling me something that I already knew to be true, but it was still advice that I needed to hear, and will probably need to hear again. Making an actionable plan to solve whatever my current crisis happens to be works 100% better than just hoping it will resolve itself. Even if it is a crisis that I am incapable of solving by myself  it does make me feel better to have checked off a to-do list of boxes so I can show myself proof that I have done all I can. Checklists, writing out a plan, all of the things that you see the very organized people automatically doing...it helps!

If there is anything to say about hope, it is not a plan, and it takes a team. In both scenarios, where hope was viable and where it was not, I had people that I could depend on. I might not have known it at the time of my worst crisis, but they were there all the same.  My mental health journey is a journey I could not do alone. I learned through trial and error that if it takes more than one person to steal the Death Star plans, or win the Champions League, or design a rocket...then it might be helpful to have a group of people to count on, or as I have been calling it throughout the book: your circle.

## Chapter 11: The Riverbend: Finding Joy Now

When you are struggling with a mental illness, the hope for an abstract and "somewhere" better future is necessary and also a trap. While we need to keep focused on a better tomorrow it is a challenge not to get stuck in the mindset that only tomorrow will be better. Today is worth something too.

Oftentimes, my partner and I go hiking. We love the outdoors and do our best to experience nature as much as we can. Hiking, backpacking, kayaking, etc. For both of us being in nature is part of how we maintain our mental health. When the world is crazy we escape into the woods.

On this particular hike I had the GPS showing how far we had left to go until we reached our destination: a beautiful waterfall.  Our route was taking us along the bank of this stunning river flowing through a forest deep in the Appalachian

Mountains. She asked me how far we had left and I answered both truthfully and choosing my words carefully:" oh, it is just around the riverbend!" As we are both children of the 90s, we could not help but sing a few lines from Disney's "Pocahontas".

As I often do while on our hikes, I tend to reflect. Nature is an amazing and freeing place and being outside in the woods is definitely a part of how I handle moments of anxiety and depression. Our short outburst into Disney sing- along caused me to think about my life and how I have been living it. Most of the accomplishments and things that I have done have been about getting to the next thing. Then the next. On and on. Happiness was always something that was forever just around the riverbend. Needless to say, that might be a contributing factor as to why I have struggled to enjoy much of life.

When I graduated high school, I felt nothing. Nothing except the coming challenge of college. This was supposed to be an achievement. In my career as a teacher I have seen many students so happy and proud to have accomplished this goal in an early part of life. Yet, looking back I felt nothing.

When I graduated college after a horrendous freshman year that included losing a scholarship and surviving a suicide attempt; joining a fraternity, making some of my best friends, joining a mental health advocacy organization, publishing a book trying to make a difference for other young people's mental health, and graduating with pretty alright grades considering; I felt nothing. Nothing but the unease at moving onto the next thing. No sense of accomplishment, just get on with it and go to the next thing. I felt I had to keep moving forward to survive.

My story with graduate school is much the same. I felt hardly any excitement about getting accepted, just in the way that it allows me to keep moving forward.  Always on to the next thing. Just keep moving forward. Landing my first career job, winning a teacher of the year award, landing my next career job...nothing, keep moving forward. I kept telling myself that my happiness was up ahead, in the future. If I could just accomplish X, Y, or Z then I would be happy.

Even non career related checkmarks felt like "okay, on to the next thing". When I finally bought a motorcycle fulfilling the dream of 10 year old me, I should have been happy. I had worked hard, saved money, and made my first adult purchase, buying the bike outright.  No doubt it was fun, but no matter, onto the next thing.

When I earned a teacher of the year award for my work, I should be happy...right? I had vindication for being good at a chosen career. No, just keep moving forward. Your happiness is in the future. This is a dangerous trap to fall into.

This mentality of never stopping to enjoy success or happy moments has been caustic. It has ruined moments I should be proud of and should have enjoyed more. Believing that happier moments, real and good moments were in the future had been a defense mechanism to my depression. Depression can't ruin the moment if I never stop to try and enjoy it, right?

It is a mentality of living in fear. Of being afraid of the present moment. By having this fantasy of an abstract tomorrow I was avoiding problems and good moments in the present. While imagining and dreaming of a better future is healthy and we all want the future to be brighter, getting lost in that mentality can mean you miss out on the joys that are present today. That is not saying every day is a joy, there are plenty of trials and tribulations. There are economic crashes, inflation, war, famine, your boss might be a jerk, you and your partner might be having a fight, your kids might be getting on your last nerve, the car breaks down, whatever. Bad is always going to happen. Good is equally going to happen too. You have to be open to seeing the good in your present as well as your future. Happiness is right now, not just around the riverbend.

# Chapter 12: The Golden Rule

Growing up in a church culture in the Southeastern United States, you hear a lot about the "Golden Rule". It is drilled into you in Sunday School, elementary school teachers use it to remind their charges not to be jerks to one another, and it seems to be the advice that the older generations default to.

The "Golden Rule" is "treat others the way you would like to be treated". You wouldn't want to be treated as less than or unworthy, so why treat others that way? It is a good rule to have in your life. While it does not explicitly say it, it is heavily implied that the way you treat others will reflect back on you. Essentially a much less advanced idea of karma. As I assume most people want to be treated with real respect and truly valued as people, it is a good rule for our society as a whole and for our interpersonal interactions. If we are all abiding by the Golden Rule then you can imagine the polite and fair society that follows. It sounds like a dream or a utopia, and I imagine many of the people reading this would not mind a world where everyone was treated fairly. I also have an amendment to the Golden Rule: treat yourself as you wish others treated you.   In the case of mental health though, the Golden Rule and its amendment are rarely applied.

The COVID-19 pandemic brought the world to a screeching halt. Then, much like a person learning to drive a manual car, a bunch of lurches and stalls before everything got started again. This halt and multiple lurches and stalls affected everyone in all walks of life around the world. Industries shut down, we shut ourselves inside and increased the time spent staring at screens, interpersonal relationships were sidelined. At the start of the pandemic I lived alone in faculty housing at a suddenly empty boarding school.

I did not physically touch another person for three

months and hardly saw anyone face to face. Even for

those who never got sick or did not have a loss in the

family, the shutting down of the world and clouds of

fear, uncertainty and doubt made life that much

more difficult.

As the world started to try and get itself back

into first gear with more than a few lurches and

stalls, some well meaning people began proselytizing

about mental health and how everyone's mental

health had collectively gone down the toilet during

2020. There were industry wide calls for better

mental health services, and my field of education was

no different. We listened to hours of people telling us

about how we needed to make a better mental health

environment for our students, and of course for

ourselves.  As mentioned earlier, many references

were made to the classic airline oxygen mask safety speech and that is one that I know was a cross industry standard.

I have been fortunate to be working in the mental health advocacy space for the better part of a decade. Be it writing books, giving talks, assisting fundraisers and whatnot, it is a space near and dear to my heart. I am always appreciative of stated intentions to improve an environment's mental health. However, over the years, and especially these last few years, my enthusiasm for those in charge calling for "better mental health" has dampened. Those in charge would bring in a person who usually had a good talk and would share some insightful stuff, usually including the oxygen mask story, to state that you need to take better care of yourself. It is true, it is hard to take care of the needs of others;be they clients, students, or colleagues, if you are not in a good place yourself. This talk with good intention was usually followed by a company leader saying that there would be some sort of physical fitness initiative offered very early in the morning before you had any work obligations.

Okay, great. I am thrilled that places want to see employees' lives improve, but you just wasted an hour of your "sacred" company time lecturing me about how I can use my own time to make my mental health better, while you just made my to do list longer because of this meeting that took away my working time. If institutions and corporations truly valued your mental health, they would do the hard work of internally examining how they can improve their processes to make more time for their employees to work on their mental health, not shoving it over to add one more thing to your personal time.

While mental health is very much a personal issue, and you should value it along with your physical health and take the time to see to it yourself, you are at work or in a classroom for about 1/3rd of your time. Some more, some less. Even if you are thinking about employees or students as parts of your whole grand machine, would you rather your fuel injectors be clean and operating at top capacity? Or gunked up and causing a loss of potential power and a less than peak performing engine? You of course want the best and most efficiently operating "part".

To have those best and most efficiently operating pieces and parts, it is important to treat those who look to you for guidance and leadership as you would like to be treated by someone above you. No one likes a tyrant. Sure, you can be tough and demanding, much like Sir Alex Ferguson managed top English soccer team Manchester United or Pep Guardiola at Manchester City, Bayern or Barcelona. They also go to bat for their players. They defend them and make space for them when necessary. The golden rule.

Good leaders also set an example by acting how they want their charges to act. If you intentionally make time for your mental health and let others see as such, you encourage them to do it as well.  If you are in a position of power or authority then I highly encourage you to govern by the golden rule and its amendment. Set an example: treat yourself and your mental health how you wished authority figures prior to you treated you. Also treat those beneath you with the same grace and real care that you wish prior authority figures did for you. If you are a teacher, manager, C-suite, coach, anyone in charge of other humans, you owe it to yourself and your people to do better for your and their mental

health.

## Chapter 13: Balance In All Things: Your Circle

A warlord stands over a small child in the bombed out and still burning ruins of her city. His army has just sacked the town, and in the chaos the young girl was separated from her mother. As the warlord's soldiers randomly filter the captured survivors of their invasion into two columns, he speaks pleasantly and softly to the young girl, taking her to the side. Pulling out a small knife, he balances it on his pointer finger. "Perfectly balanced, as all things should be. Too much to one side or the other..." he states as he wobbles the knife back and forth. He hands the knife to the young girl "Here, you try." as if on cue his death squads open fire on one of the columns of prisoners. When the smoke clears, the other surviving column of prisoners is released to live their lives in peace. Perfectly balanced, as all things should be.

This story comes from Marvel's *Avengers: Infinity War* where the ultimate bad guy that they have spent 20 movies building towards, Thanos, is on a misguided quest to "save" the galaxy. In his eyes the universe is being overrun. The population across all star systems of all forms of life is too high and everyone is on a collision course with a resource crisis. His wildly unpopular solution is the "fair" random genocide of half of the universes' population. All to eventually be completed with a simple snap of his fingers using the mystical and insanely powerful Infinity Stones. If only all problems could be solved with a snap.

The concept of balance is just as true in life, physics, and in relationships. To tip a scale, one must add or remove a weight. To receive your coffee at Starbucks, you must give the barista $5. To move your car forward you must drain its fuel source. As said in the science fiction movie *Interstellar:* "The only way humans have figured out how to move forward is by leaving something behind."

When it comes to building your circle this lesson from physics or supervillains about balance is crucially important. Your goal should be to build a circle of people around you that is willing to help, willing to listen, willing to work to help you overcome. A positive community that wants to see you become your best self. To achieve this goal, you have to be willing to give it as well.

Building a trusting and caring community around you is hard work, and it can be very tough to do if you are already in a dark mental spot. On some level we are all "selfish". Not necessarily a bad trait, you just need to ensure that your biological and physical needs are met. When it comes to building a circle of people that you trust enough to help unburden your problems, the temptation can be to simply unload. To use the other person like a mental dumpster. Unfortunately this is not sustainable nor does it create healthy relationships.

To build a real and lasting relationship with someone you trust, where you both can discuss problems, emotions, and feelings in a safe and respectable environment requires you both to bring balance. This is where the work is hard. It could mean that even when your problems seem insurmountable, you also have to be willing to listen to your friends and validate their struggles, and help them overcome them.

This is even harder in a moment of need or crisis. You have to be willing to help your circle find their path forward. You can't gain something without giving something in return. That isn't wrong, in fact it is healthy. Relying on people without being available for them to rely on you makes you, frankly, a leech. Draining others without ever letting them give back.

Relationships, no matter how long they have existed, can become tough to bear when one party only takes. When one party asks for a listening ear and sound advice, but then can't or won't return the favor. This is a trap that many people fall into when trying to build a trusting circle, and it is not always out of malice. It can be incredibly hard to be empathetic and think of others when your own mind has turned on you and you are desperately grasping for life lines.It is a trap that leads to many men feeling even more alone in the midst of their deepest crisis. This can lead to many lost or damaged relationships, feelings of abandonment, and a propensity to lean into causes or coping mechanisms that are not good for anyone.

I actively encourage everyone to consciously take a moment and check in on their circle, especially if you are a person who is always looking to lean on them for assistance. The act of checking in on your friends can go a long way in building the two way street of support that is the foundation of a healthy relationship.

A healthy relationship also has boundaries. Sometimes your friends might not have the mental space to handle the exchange required to hear you out, and that is something you have to be okay with. Having your own boundaries and knowing yourself is healthy too. If you definitely do not believe you are capable of being an active and helpful listener to your circle, tell them! Saying "no, I am unable to help right now" is just as important as offering a helping hand. By the same token, you have to be willing to hear that from your circle as well. A "I can't right now" does not mean the relationship is over, or that they/ you are never willing to be a shoulder to lean on again. It is healthy and can even help lead to a much more balanced exchange in the relationship. Trust, open and honest communication, and the setting of boundaries are the key ingredients of building your circle.

Maintaining a balance in your relationships is required for a healthy circle to be built around you and for you to be an active and healthy part of other's circles. You should strive to have a balance on your time, empathy, and emotional load. If friends only ever call you to borrow your truck to move their couches, then it is not a balanced relationship. You wouldn't be okay with just being a free moving service, so you and everyone should not be okay with being a free emotional mover either. Finding a way to strike a balance is the key to building healthy relationships and ensuring the continuing care and

longevity of your circle.

# Chapter 14: Echoes in Eternity; Building Your Legacy

A pilot, two teachers, and a carpenter are sitting around a bonfire...while this is probably the setup to a great joke, I am afraid I don't have the punchline for it. Talking around a fire is a time honored and quintessential "manly" tradition. In my experience it is those times when we are the most vulnerable and the most real with each other. As is the case with the people listed above, we sat around fires and talked for hours on end. Topics ranged from societal issues and how we in our infinite wisdom would solve them, sports, pop culture, religion, personal problems, relationship trouble, and a common one: legacy. How would we want to be remembered after we have gone on from this world?

Thinking about one's legacy is a natural part of life. It tends to be brought to the forefront during times of change or when forced to confront our own mortality. For those of us, like myself, who struggle with suicidal thoughts and ideation it can be a very sobering thought process. It was not until a few years after my attempt at suicide when I thought about how I would be remembered. I would have been just another sad story of some 18 year old who couldn't hack it, or some unfortunate example of a person who "fell through the cracks". To my parents I would forever be their little boy, who they viewed as having boundless potential that I would never fulfill. There probably would have been candlelight vigils and whatnot. Would the attendees have known me? Would they have actually cared?

I have unfortunately seen a few friends and acquaintances lose their battles with suicide. Much like I described above; they are remembered for who they were, and sadly who they could have been. Their legacy is one of what was and what could have been.

Looking back 9 years on from my attempt and I am thankful that I failed.

Some of us are going to struggle our whole lives with our illness. Fighting depression, anxiety, bipolar, or any mental illness. Some people are fortunate and therapy or medicine fixes their issue in a relatively short amount of time and through a lot of hard work.  Others are less so and have to settle in for the long haul, a space I find myself occupying currently. There is always that darkness waiting to creep back in. That panic looking for a crack in the armor. I still expect to live a full and happy life! I just know that there will always be an element of struggle.

The passing of famous and high profile  people by suicide such as Kurt Cobain, Anthony Bourdain, or Naomi Judd brings the issue to the forefront of everyone's minds. It shows that everyone, no matter their level of success, age, or lifestyle can be subject to the ravages of a mental health problem.

Using the people above as examples; their incredible lives makes their death all the more sad and further proves to everyone that mental health is a war. Not a battle that has a definite end, but a war that lasts as long as it needs to. I choose to draw strength in these moments and double down. Their end is not how I want my war to end. That is not how I want to be remembered.

I don't know how my story will end, will I be taken out by some despot starting World War Three? A car crash? Cancer? I can't possibly know, but I don't want it to be by my own hand. Coming to that realization took many years of working and constant maintenance work. If you get nothing else from this book, know that mental health is hard work!

As the fictional but inspiring gladiator and general Maximus said "what we do in life echoes in eternity." I want my echo to be one of positivity, hope, and strength. Both for myself, and hopefully for those I have had the honor of being a part of their lives. What do you want your echo to be? Believe in it and it will be so.

# Chapter 15: I Am Worthy

Axios is a mindset. It is something that you have to believe in every fiber of your being: I am worthy. You are worthy. We are worthy.

Men are worthy of being able to safely and confidently discuss their emotions and feelings without shame for having them. Men are worthy of better responses to our legitimate problems than "suck it up" or "be a man". Men are worthy of being freed from the oppression of extremist and unhealthy ideologies that do nothing but drive us apart and make us feel worse.  Men are worthy of coming along on the journey to break the stigma around mental health. Men are worthy of having our stories heard and listened to.

You are worthy. You are worthy of a life where you do not have to be afraid of the feelings and emotions that you have. You are worthy of having the ability to tell someone honestly "I am not okay" and have that received at face value and with respect and dignity. You are worthy of building a world around you that accepts you for you. That respects you when you have off days. You are worthy of silencing that voice in your head that tells you "you can't succeed". You are worthy of finding a foothold to arrest your downward slide and begin your rise again. You are worthy of a job and career that values you as a human as much as it does for your labor or your skills, because you cannot have one without the other. You are worthy of having a supportive circle around you, and of being included in others supportive circles. You are worthy of being remembered for your deeds. You are worthy.

Axios is a mindset. It takes a shift in thinking. It takes an effort to maintain that work and that way of thought. It is not without setbacks. There are challenges and there will be moments when you stumble and have a crisis. Where you might feel you are not worthy. Keep the flame alive inside you, and remember that you are worthy.  Above all, Axios is mostly reliant on you. It is up to you to reframe your mind to the one you know you are worthy of having. It is up to you to build your life around you to the one you know you are worthy of. It is up to you to surround yourself with supportive and loving people, and it is up to you to love and support those who support you. Axios is a lot of work. Believe in the work. Hard work. Know that you are worthy.

Axios- I am worthy.

Thank you for taking the time to read this book. It is my hope that you learned something, are inspired, or that it has helped you find peace.

If you would like to follow my writing further, I publish a Men's Mental Health related blog: Average Joe's Mental Health. You can find it linked in the QR Code below.

Again, thank you for reading and Axios.